LOVE VEGAN

How to Look 10 Years Younger

DISCLAIMER

'How to Look 10 Years Younger' does not provide medical advice and nothing contained herein shall be construed as medical advice. The full contents of the book are for informational purposes only. The information is not intended to diagnose, treat, cure or prevent any illnesses or diseases.

'How to Look 10 Years Younger' does not provide specific information or advice regarding skin intolerance or allergies. It is the responsibility of the reader to ensure any diagnosed or potential allergens or intolerances are identified and excluded from the advice and recipes.

The author and publisher make no guarantee as to the availability of ingredients mentioned in this book. The author cannot be held responsible for any recipe not working. The author and publisher will take no responsibility for any issues arising when using the recipes within the book. It is the reader's responsibility to take the proper precautions and ensure ingredients are suitable for their skin. Tell your doctor immediately if any side effects occur from using the creams or masks within the book.

The author and publisher take no responsibility for any liability, loss or damage caused as a result of use of the information within this book.

Every effort has been made to prepare this material to ensure it's accuracy, however the author nor publisher will be held responsible if there is information deemed as inaccurate or deemed to be misused.

CONTENTS

FOREWORD

Everything in life is a matter of choices. Every single day we are faced with situations that require us to make privy choices and perhaps those that are most important are those concerning our health, beauty, and skin care.

You may have wrongly assumed that there's nothing much you can do to improve your skin, get rid of premature aging or get a silky smooth supple and radiant complexion but that is so far from the truth. By making the right beauty and skin care choices, you are equipping your skin with all the ammunition it needs to fight blemishes, dryness, wrinkles, drooping, and dullness.

Of all the basic tenets of our life, beauty and skin care ranks first and in this book we are going to look at everything that you have been doing that is working well for your skin; everything that you need to stop doing immediately and a few tips and tricks to restore your fountain of youth. So sit back, it is time to floor the pedal to the metal!

INTRODUCTION

Growing up, I was always the girl who looked six years younger than all the other girls in the class which actually bothered me at the time. My mom always told me to enjoy the fountain of youth as there would come a time when I would wish I looked ten years younger.

My mom was always very gentle on her skin and she would apply all sorts of weird masks at night but I always loved how radiant her skin was. Aside from how to apply makeup, I also picked up quite a number of tricks to keep my face and skin always looking beautiful.

One thing that I vividly remember is the kind of foods we ate growing up. Fruits and vegetables always formed the largest portion of our meals and I remember battling my mum to allow me to carry pretzels to school like most of the kids, but all I got was a fruit salad or veggies.

Fast forward to date and I am so grateful for all the amazing things I was able to learn from my mom and I want to share them all with you so that you too can have beautiful skin. I cannot emphasize enough the importance of a healthy diet, and we are going to look at how this impacts your skin in the book.

The theme of this book is to make use of what Mother Nature has endowed us with and not to always go to the cosmetic counter for the latest beauty invention. Mother Nature always knows best!

WHAT CAUSES THE SKIN TO AGE?

There are countless things that causes our skin to age. Some we can influence but others we cannot do anything about. For instance, we cannot change the natural aging process and this plays a key role in causing our skin to age.

It is very natural for our skin to lose some of its youthful glow and with time, we all get some visible lines on our face. Our genetic makeup largely controls when we start noticing our skin becoming drier and thinner. But, we are going to look at very effective ways of slowing down the skin aging process as we progress in the book.

However, aside from the natural aging process, here are the major culprits responsible for aging your skin:

SMOKING

Did you know that a single puff of cigarette smoke emits approximately 40,000 free radicals? These free radicals deplete your body of vitamin C and thus accelerate the aging process.

SLEEPLESS NIGHTS

Beauty sleep is so aptly named as this is the time your body recovers from the strenuous day's activities. Additionally, sleep helps regulate the secretion of chemicals and hormones that are responsible for immunity and vitality.

Lack of adequate sleep causes an imbalance of these vital hormones as your body is forced to be in 'active mode' when it should actually be resting. The result? Your immunity is compromised, allowing pathogens into your system.

Remember, your skin is a mirror image of your overall health and so a compromised immunity will manifest as dull skin, stress lines, slack pores, and general tissue damage.

EXCESSIVE FITNESS

We all know that keeping fit helps regulate circulation and the inflow of oxygen into your skin cells, giving you a beautiful and radiant glow. But did you also know that too much exercise can have the complete opposite effect?

Too much exercise triggers your body to produce reactive oxygen, which can become too much for our natural antioxidant defense. As a result, your body starts extracting antioxidants from your tissues to counter the reactive oxygen. In the end, your skin is left dry and damaged.

NUTRITION

Show me your skin and I will be able to tell you what you eat. If you are constantly snacking on junk food then your skin is going to look like junk. If you regularly indulge in antioxidant rich foods, your skin is going to be the true picture of health and the ultimate fountain of youth.

Later on, we are going to look at the perfect 'skin foods'.

TOO MUCH SUN

Who doesn't like a good summer tan? But, before you get into your bikini and hit the beach, you should know that sun exposure is the number one culprit when it comes to brown spots, wrinkles, slack skin, dry skin...I could go on and on. Do not be seduced by the lure of a beautiful bronzed tan and forget the negative implications it could have on your skin.

Use collagen-rich sunscreen creams and most of all, stay away from the scorching sun at peak times!

Now that we know what's been keeping us from smooth, supple skin, let us now look at the most effective anti-aging ingredients.

WHAT ARE THE BEST ANTI-AGING INGREDIENTS?

Before we get into the ingredients you should apply on your skin to restore your youthful glow, it is important to emphasize that your diet is going to have a profound effect on how your skin looks. Treat your body like a temple and eat whole, natural foods that are going to supply your skin with essential nutrients that will keep it healthy and radiant.

Here are the top five anti-aging ingredients:

RETINOL

There is a reason why retinol is referred to as the cure-all when it comes to your skin. It is highly endowed with vitamin A and it is the best solution for wrinkles, sagging skin, fine stress lines, dullness and sun spots. So, in short, this is one of the best anti-aging ingredients around.

Who is it for:

It is best suited for anyone aged 30 and above.

How does it work?

The vitamin A in retinol speeds up the growth of new cells and the elimination of dead cells thus leaving you with clear skin. It also boosts elastin and collagen which help stimulate cell repair at the deepest skin level. To top it all, retinol increases blood vessel formation thus improving circulation of blood into all your cells leaving you with youthful, radiant skin.

How to make it work best?

Start by washing your face with warm water then apply retinol, with your skin still damp. It works best in the dark so always apply it right before you go to sleep. Wash your face in the morning and treat your skin to an organic moisturizer.

COLLAGEN

Collagen is the ultimate skin toner. This protein is usually found in marine life or in animal connective tissue and since it is non-water soluble, it helps the skin to hold its natural water thus giving you a soft and plumped up look.

Who is it for?

Everyone

How does it work?

Collagen acts like a cushion for your skin. It helps improve elasticity thus giving you a fresh and silky smooth appearance. In addition, it keeps our skin strong and healthy from the retention of the skin's moisture.

How to make it work best?

Collagen molecules are much larger than skin cells and thus cannot penetrate through. To get the actual benefits of collagen, it is best ingested. You can obtain collagen supplements or better yet, you can eat collagen rich foods such as egg whites, wheat germ, bone broth and wild caught fish.

VITAMIN C (L-ASCORBIC ACID)

This is a super ingredient that not only helps boost your immunity but it also makes your skin supple. However, many skin care products contain unstable vitamin C that won't actually do much for your skin. Look for L-ascorbic acid on the ingredients as this is the stable form of vitamin C.

Who is it for?

Anyone from age 25 and above

How does it work?

This is a powerful antioxidant that reduces inflammation, helps build collagen (including dermal collagen that reduces wrinkles) and that also produces elasticity leaving you with glowing plumped up skin.

How to make it work best?
Apply it on damp skin so it penetrates deeper into your skin cells.

You can also eat vitamin C rich foods such as citrus fruits, broccoli, dark leafy greens, guava, brussel sprouts and camu camu.

VITAMIN E

In a few words, vitamin E is a skin healing powerhouse. This is the best ingredient to use to reverse collagen destruction, dryness, stress lines and wrinkles.

Who is it for?
Anyone looking to rejuvenate their skin

How does it work?
Vitamin E neutralizes free radicals that damage skin cells and it also helps strengthen the skin barrier thus boosting immunity. This explains why vitamin E oil works effectively for scars, burns, cuts and even cracked cuticles.

How to make it work best?
Wash your face with warm water and mild soap then apply your product. Leave it on all night so it can heal your skin from inside. Rinse your face in the morning and apply a mild moisturizer.

You can use the liquid from within a capsule and puncture it using a needle to release the vitamin E. It is recommended that for best results use vitamin E within a homemade face cream - please see recipes within the book.

If you are taking vitamin E supplements, follow the prescribed advice.

ANTIOXIDANTS

Antioxidants are better known as 'the skin fixers'. In a nutshell, antioxidants protect your skin cells from environmental damage.

Who is it for?

Everyone!

How do they work?

Antioxidants go deep into your skin where they convert harmful free radicals that are responsible for aging your skin into harmless compounds. This action stops free radicals from damaging elastin, collagen, and DNA.

How to make them work best?

For cosmetic antioxidants, go with a serum as they tend to penetrate the skin better compared to creams. Additionally, opt for a blend as each antioxidant targets specific free radicals thus will make the protection more potent.

For nutritional antioxidants, here is a simple guideline:

Vitamin A: Carrots, spinach, kale, pumpkin, cantaloupe and liver.

Vitamin C: Broccoli, camu camu, Brussels sprouts, citrus fruits and guava.

Vitamin E: Tomatoes, olive and walnut oils, wheat germ oil, carrots, and oats.

Bioflavonoids: Citrus fruits, onions, berries, red wine and sea buckthorn.

Polyphenols: Dark chocolate, green tea, berries, peanuts, walnuts and pomegranates.

WHAT ARE THE BEST NATURAL ANTI-AGING OILS?

Mother Nature has always provided us with the best skin care products. If you are looking for something that is free from synthetic fragrances and parabens and that deeply penetrates your skin layers to rejuvenate it, look no further than what nature has provided us with – natural oils.

Are natural oils better than creams?

In one word – YES!

Natural oils are directly absorbed into your skin and thus work on your skin from inside. Creams, on the other hand, consist of water, wax, and an emulsifier. The wax and emulsifier make the cream sit on the surface of the skin and doesn't really penetrate through the skin.

Whether your skin is oily, dry, sensitive or mature, here are some good natural oils that will help restore and rejuvenate your skin.

COCONUT OIL

Coconut oil is nature's very own sunscreen. This natural oil works better that the artificial and overly-processed sunscreens that are laden with additives and chemicals.

Coconut oil contains saturated fats that retain the moisture content of your skin, keeping it smooth and supple. This natural oil also contains capric, lauric and caprylic fatty acids that have very strong and effective antimicrobial and disinfectant properties. It is therefore very effective when applied on open wounds as it helps the skin heal faster.

Coconut is also well endowed with vitamin E and essential proteins that help repair your skin tissue and also keep your skin healthy and radiant. Additionally, coconut oil is also one of the most popular natural anti-aging solutions.

All you need to do is clean your face with warm water and mild soap, pat gently using a towel to remove excess water, then gently rub coconut oil all over your skin and sit back as you reap all the coconut oil benefits.

MORINGA OIL

This natural oil is extracted from the seeds of a tree known as the moringa oleifera tree commonly referred to as the horseradish tree or drumstick tree.

This oil is well known for its cleansing, moisturizing and emollient properties. It is very easily absorbed into your skin thereby improving your skin's radiance and general appearance. Moringa oil is also jam-packed with vitamins A, C and E.

Moringa oil deeply moisturizes your skin offering relief to dry skin, eczema, dermatitis and psoriasis. It is also highly endowed with antioxidants that fight off free radicals, leading to premature aging and the formation of wrinkles. Moringa oil also contains hormones that promote skin cell growth thus repairing damaged tissues and delaying aging.

It's high vitamin C content helps stabilize collagen and thus reduces fine lines as well as stress lines leaving you with smooth, supple and radiant skin.

OLIVE OIL

You probably have olive oil as a staple in your pantry but have you ever thought of it as a beauty powerhouse? Not only is olive oil one of the best makeup removers, it is also very rich in vitamin E, giving your skin a youthful and healthy glow and thus qualifying it as nature's own anti-aging 'cream'.

Having dryness problems? Well, olive oil is a very gentle and effective moisturizer. Use a cotton ball to directly apply olive oil on your skin and wait for your skin to plump up beautifully.

If you suffer from dry, inflamed or itchy skin, that is usually a sign of skin conditions such as eczema, dermatitis or psoriasis. Instead of spending a lot of money on store bought creams, rub some olive oil on the problem areas for instant relief.

Did you know that olive oil is nature's very own shaving cream? If after shaving with water and soap you experience razor rash, it's about time you started using olive oil. Due to its moisturizing properties, olive oil will leave you with a very smooth shave. All you need to do is coat your skin with olive oil before you shave.

ROSEHIP SEED OIL

This oil is derived from the 'fruit' of the rose and is highly enriched with antioxidants including lycopene and beta-carotene. As it is also a very good source of vitamins A and C, rosehip seed oil protects your skin from premature aging.

This oil contains essential fatty acids that helps repair skin tissue and also regenerates your skin cells as well as aiding with the formation of collagen.

This natural oil is very effective in treating dermatitis, scars, uneven skin tone, stretch marks, fine lines and acne scarring. Rosehip oil works by moisturizing the dry areas of your skin and is easily absorbed thereby making it a great moisturizer for all skin types.

AVOCADO OIL

We all love the creamy goodness of the avocado fruit but did you also know that it is a hidden beauty treasure!

Mashing up an avocado and spreading it on your face can be quite a messy affair but certainly worth your efforts as the vitamins in an avocado have powerful anti-aging properties.

Try out some of the lovely avocado based face masks later in the book, or just add some to a salad if you prefer to reap the benefits by eating them. Avocados aren't only an effective skin care product, but they are also very convenient to use as you can purchase them inexpensively from your local supermarket.

Avocado oil is packed with vitamins A, D and E, disease-fighting antioxidants, essential proteins and fats and potassium. All these ingredients, when combined, leave you with smooth, supple, radiant and strong skin.

Avocado oil is a great moisturizer and provides relief for dry and inflamed skin. Additionally, you can use it to clear a scaly scalp and also relieve itchiness. This wonder oil also helps boost collagen production, which not only gives you a youthful glow, but it also reduces the effects of aging leaving your skin beautifully plumped up.

WHAT IF I DON'T LIKE APPLYING OIL ON MY SKIN?

Not to worry. All these oils can be ingested and they will still offer your skin the same benefits. However, if you have a wound or lesion, it is best to dab a little oil using a cotton ball on the problem area. Otherwise, you can always add a few teaspoons of natural oils to your salad or smoothies for maximum benefits.

Avoid denaturing essential nutrients by cooking the oils, aim to eat them in their raw forms.

ANTI-AGING SUPERFOODS

Earlier on we looked at the effects your diet has on the condition of your skin – we even mentioned that if you show me your skin and I will tell you how healthy your diet is!

Well, we are now going to delve deeper into 9 of the most powerful superfoods that are literally going to reverse the aging process and give you the most beautiful, radiant and supple skin that you have always desired.

AVOCADOS

We looked at the benefits of avocado oil in the previous section and now we are going to look at why you should be eating more and more avocados.

Avocados have a special and healthy type of fat – monounsaturated fat that helps keep your skin hydrated round the clock. The monounsaturated fat also helps your body absorb vitamins and other nutrients better, thus providing your skin with all essential nutrients.

Wondering how to eat avocado? Swap your mayo and other fatty salad dressings with avocado. It is natural, creamy and adds a great punch of flavor to your food. Yum!

CINNAMON

Adding just a tablespoon of cinnamon to your food every day will improve your skin tone. It is a good source of fiber that helps eliminate accumulated waste products. By doing so, cinnamon helps flush out toxins that would otherwise clog your skin.

Cinnamon is a very versatile spice that can be added to virtually all foods. It is always best to eat it raw. Try adding cinnamon powder to your smoothies, porridge or yoghurt which will, in turn, help you fight off free radicals.

Additionally, cinnamon contains antimicrobial and antibacterial properties that will help keep your skin healthy and clear. Ingested cinnamon also helps boost collagen production making it one of the best anti-aging ingredients.

Make cinnamon tea by boiling cinnamon powder in water and adding a bit of honey for immense health benefits for your skin and overall well-being.

BERRIES

Who knew that these tiny fruits are jam-packed with beauty goodness? Not only are they tasty, but they are also infused with powerful anti-aging and skin toning benefits. Choose berries that are rich in color such as deep purple, red and black as this is an indicator of the large amounts of antioxidants that they contain.

Due to their high antioxidant levels, berries are great at fighting off free radicals that cause wrinkling, premature aging and skin tissue degeneration, providing you with healthy and supple skin. The great thing about berries is that they are very versatile and you can just pop them in your mouth as a snack, make a yummy smoothie, and use them to make a salad.

Whichever way you decide to eat them, ensure you get a serving of these beauty-packed berries every day and you won't need to worry about your skin looking dull or gaining weight. Berries have a high fiber content with very little sugar, so in essence they help your body eliminate waste and toxins, leaving your skin clear and radiant.

NUTS

We all love nuts because they are the perfect healthy snack when hunger pangs start setting in, but did you know that when eaten in moderation nuts can do wonders for your skin?

These tasty treats are endowed with fiber, healthy fats and protein that not only make your skin radiant and stronger, but they also help get rid of waste material and toxins from your body, leaving you with clear skin that is free of toxic burden.

They also help with the formation of collagen that allows your skin to rejuvenate from deep inside, healing any damaged tissues. This combined with the fatty acids works to eliminate wrinkles, stress and fine lines.

Additionally, nuts are very rich in vitamins and minerals and helping get rid of blemishes and brown spots. So next time you are looking for a mid-day snack, go for a handful of nuts and nourish your skin from within.

COCONUT

This tropical fruit has immense benefits when it comes to your skin. From coconut water to its white flesh and silky oil, every component of this fruit apart from the hard shell is good for your skin.

Coconuts contain monounsaturated fats that work wonders on your complexion. These fats lock-in the moisture in your skin and smooths it at the same time. The result? Baby-smooth, supple and extra radiant skin. Who doesn't want to have skin as smooth as a baby's?

You can use coconut oil to cook your food and you can also apply it on your skin overnight after a shower to allow it to work its magic all through the night. Regular ingestion and application of coconut oil on your skin will take care of any marks, blemishes and stretch marks.

Additionally the fiber from the white flesh of coconuts helps your body eliminate waste and toxic material thereby restoring your youthful good looks.

FISH AND FISH OILS

We know that fish and fish oil supplements promote heart health, joint health and eye health but, did you also know that they also promote skin health? Fish and fish oil contain special fatty acids that are not produced by our bodies but are essential for a healthy and glowing skin.

The omega 3 fats found in fish, trigger a positive inflammatory response that makes your skin clearer and more radiant. Again, these fatty acids are some of the best natural moisturizers that revitalize your skin from inside out giving a very fresh look.

Look for wild caught fish as they have the lowest instances of mercury contamination such as anchovies, sardines, salmon and albacore tuna. Swordfish, shark, tilefish and king mackerel have a very high mercury content and should be avoided.

TURMERIC

This spice of beauty has been used for centuries thanks to the long list of benefits that it offers to the skin. This is one of the few cure all ingredients for the skin. From healing and hydrating dry skin, treating acne spots, keeping your skin supple and improving pigmentation to providing you with sun protection, turmeric should be a staple in your pantry as well as beauty cabinet.

You can make turmeric tea by adding a teaspoon of turmeric to two cups of boiling water and adding honey to taste. This simple recipe will help your skin heal from within if taken on a regular basis. You can also add turmeric to nearly all of your meals, giving it a rich color.

You can use turmeric to make a paste using milk or yogurt to act as a facial mask and an exfoliator. Whichever way you chose to have it, the bottom line is your skin is going to thank you.

HONEY

Raw honey is one of the best foods you can use to nourish your skin. Not only does it have a hefty serving of antioxidants that deeply nourish your skin, it is also endowed with antibacterial properties that heal your complexion and restore your natural glow.

Honey also helps clear your pores leaving them very clear and radiant. It also does a very good job of treating acne due to its antibacterial properties.

If you are looking for a complexion boost and something to protect your skin from premature aging, honey is one of your best bets!

APPLE CIDER VINEGAR

We use this to add a punch to our raw salads but did you also know that it has amazing benefits for your skin? Why should you apply such a smelly liquid on your face when there are millions of beautifully scented products that you can douse your face in?

Well, the answer is quite simple, if you want smooth, supple, blemish free and glowing skin, then you should use apple cider to clean your face, as well as adding it to your food.

This wonder vinegar is made from fermented apples. The fermentation process releases healthy enzymes that are loaded with antioxidants as well as antibacterial properties, and adding this vinegar to your food or beverages allows your body to heal your skin from within.

Additionally, washing your face with apple cider vinegar will help take care of all your blemish problems - just remember to do this on a regular basis for best results.

WORST FOODS FOR YOUR SKIN

By now, we have established that certain nutrients can work wonders for your skin. It is also true that certain foods can wreck havoc on your skin, leaving you with aged, patchy, dry and scarred skin.

Here are five foods that you should avoid like the plague:

PROCESSED FOODS

Our supermarkets today are laden with over-processed junk foods that are doused in additives, chemicals and preservatives. French fries, candy, white bread and sugar will spike your blood sugar levels. This action confuses your hormones, triggering them to initiate excessive oil production which clogs your pores and prematurely ages your skin. Opt for whole natural foods that have all their nutrients intact.

SHELLFISH

Lobster, crab and shrimp are very high in iodine which can clog your pores and even spike an acne breakout. Swap shellfish for a healthier option that will do amazing things to your skin, such as wild caught fish which are endowed with omega 3 fatty acids.

CAFFEINE

A regular intake of caffeinated drinks dehydrates you, which negatively impacts your skin's collagen and elasticity. In time this leads to wrinkles and sagging, aging you by years. To avoid this, replace your morning coffee with a big glass of water and even add a dash of lemon juice for more flavor. Regular water intake hydrates your skin leaving it supple and moisturized from within.

AGAVE

This is deemed to be one of the best sugar substitutes available but unfortunately, it packs too much fructose for your skin to handle. Fructose is digested in your liver and it usually breaks down collagen faster compared to regular sugar. If you don't want crow's feet on your eyes, then keep away from agave.

MILK

This is a breakfast staple for many households but unless you are consuming milk from grass fed animals, then you are better off avoiding milk. Cows are constantly fed with produce that contain growth hormones, and milk may still carry these hormones even after pasteurization.

After digestion, when these hormones get into your bloodstream, then can trigger excessive oil production, clogging up your pores in the process and even causing a skin breakout. Try milk substitutes instead such as almond, coconut or soy milk.

The list is endless for foods that can damage your skin but a good rule of thumb is to eat foods that are whole and natural and that grow as a plant as opposed to those that are made in a plant!

SPECIFIC PROBLEM AREAS AND HOW TO COMBAT WRINKLES

Unfortunately wrinkles are an unavoidable part of aging. However, this does not mean that there are not proven ways to reduce the appearance and prevent the onset of more wrinkles forming.

There are times when we wake up and look in the mirror only to see your skin looking dull, grey and lifeless. Here are some tips that will target specific problem areas and help you look your best in the shortest time possible.

DARK CIRCLES UNDER YOUR EYES

Here are a few methods to instantly reduce dark circles:

- Cut two slices from a cucumber and place each on top of your eyes extending to the dark circles and lie down for ten to fifteen minutes with your eyes closed.

- Wrap two ice cubes separately, using clean clothes and place this on top of your closed eyes and lie down for about fifteen minutes.

- Place two cool tea bags on top of your eyes and relax for about fifteen minutes.

- Juice two raw potatoes and apply the paste on the darkened circles for fifteen minutes then rinse it off.

These four remedies will work like magic!

CROW'S FEET, FOREHEAD WRINKLES AND SKIN TIGHTENING

The best remedy for crows feet is one that contains vitamin E. You can buy organic vitamin E creams or you can make your own home remedies using the recipes in this book. If you opt for home remedies, just buy a vitamin E capsule, poke it and apply the oil on the crow's feet.

You can also make an egg white mask that will help make the skin firm. Additionally, include foods that are rich in vitamin E in your diet so they nourish your skin from inside. For best results you must consume these foods on a regular basis.

DROOPING CHEEKS AND SAGGING NECK

The best home remedy for drooping cheeks and sagging neck is to massage your cheeks and neck using one of the natural oils we discussed earlier. Use the back of your wrist, right below your palm to gently but firmly massage these problem areas.

You should also practice sleeping on your back as this helps prevent wrinkles forming from the pressure when sleeping on your side. It is also very important to apply collagen creams on your cheeks and neck especially overnight and remember to moisturize in the morning.

WATCH YOUR DIET AND INCLUDE COLLAGEN-RICH FOODS

Our diets and what we eat has been closely linked to aging for decades and studies have proven there is a direct correlation. The foods we eat could either be strengthening our skin, making it look healthier and more toned or creating more wrinkles on a daily basis.

The important thing to remember is that changing you diet for a day or two will not make much of a difference. If you are serious about transforming your skin and reducing the appearance of wrinkles this must be a lifestyle change. By eating fresh and wholesome food everyday you are guaranteed to see results within weeks.

In a nutshell, to avoid problems with your skin and to retain your youthful tightness and glow, ensure that you drink a minimum of 8 glasses of water every day, get adequate sleep, use natural products on your face and eat a healthy and natural diet.

TAILORING YOUR APPROACH TO DIFFERENT SKIN TYPES

IN YOUR TWENTIES…

The biggest challenge most people face when in their twenties is fighting off acne or blemishes. You should look for a water-based lotion that is oil free and that contains salicylic acid so it can hydrate your skin.

Do not sleep with your makeup on and always moisturize your face in the morning and at night just before you sleep. Remember to watch what you eat and drink to prevent wrinkles forming.

Your skin will thank you for this in years to come!

IN YOUR THIRTIES…

Unfortunately we may start noticing fine lines, small wrinkles and uneven skin tone when we turn thirty. This is the time to start using retinol and natural oils that will boost collagen production. Moisturize your skin at least twice a day, in the morning and evening. Hydrate regularly, ensuring you drink a minimum of 8 glasses of water a day.

When it comes to food, opt for foods rich in vitamins A, D and E as well as those that will boost collagen production.

IN YOUR FORTIES…

This is the time we notice age spots and wrinkles setting in. What your skin needs more than anything is collagen, hydration and vitamin E. Use only natural oils and creams that will stimulate these three. Closely monitor your diet and ensure it is fully natural and endowed with nutrients so it can help repair your skin from inside.

Avoid harsh environmental conditions such as scorching heat or the freezing cold as these will punish your skin.

IN YOUR FIFTIES...

During your fifties, your hormones will begin to shift and as a result of this, your skin can get a little dry, dehydrated and more prone to fine lines. Your body will produce less natural oils which help keep your face hydrated, meaning you need to step in with a helping hand and a good moisturiser!

It is essential a good quality moisturising cream is used, and it's even more important for it to be applied at night before bed to enable your skin to regenerate.

Be sure to exfoliate once a week and for an extra moisture surge use a facemask frequently, especially one with vitamin C.

Be sure to consume foods with high levels of antioxidants as this will also help your skin renew itself.

Try to avoid hot showers and opt for one that is lukewarm. Hot water will strip the skin of essential natural oils.

TIPS AND TRICKS TO MAINTAIN HEALTHY GLOWING SKIN

SATIN PILLOWCASE

Some people say that sleeping on a satin pillowcase is vain but there are some real beauty benefits that come with sleeping on one. Cotton pillowcases, which are commonly used, can result in sleep lines on your face. With time, these small lines will grow into fully fledged wrinkles.

Satin pillowcases allow your face to easily slide up and down without causing any friction on your face. Your face will thank you later in life for this simple trick.

AVOID SUN INDOORS THROUGH WINDOWS

Most of us are only aware of the need to take sun precaution when outdoors especially during summer. However, just because you are indoors it doesn't mean that the UV rays are any less harmful. If you drive around in your car or sit by a window in your house on a regular basis without using any sunscreen, you will notice brown spots and other aging signs on your skin.

SITTING TOO CLOSE TO THE FIREPLACE

Ever heard of the toasted skin syndrome?

It's actually not a disease, rather it's a sort of rash that forms on your skin on the side that you sit closest to the fire with. It's not painful or itchy it just isn't pretty. So even on a cold night, don't sit too close to your fireplace, choose a safe distance and protect your skin with warm clothing.

EXFOLIATE AT LEAST ONCE A WEEK

This is one of the ways to instantly make your skin smooth. When you exfoliate you rid your skin of dry skin cells on the surface creating a radiant and smoother appearance.

Exfoliators help slow down the aging process so if you are worried about wrinkles, ensure you exfoliate at least once a week. Your skin will also absorb the moisturiser you choose to use much more efficiently.

DO NOT TAKE VERY HOT SHOWERS

Why is it that the best things in life are usually bad for us? Well, the same applies to hot showers. Very hot showers on a regular basis can highly dehydrate your skin leaving you with patched and dry skin. This is because your skins outer layer usually has a thin layer of oil that locks moisture in your skin. Hot showers burn off this layer allowing moisture to escape.

Opt for cool showers instead that will leave you feeling refreshed.

SLEEP ON YOUR BACK

Sleeping on your back ensures you don't get any sleep lines on your face that can later grow into wrinkles. If you are used to sleeping in the fetal position, it is going to take some getting used to but the benefits are certainly going to pay off.

DIY VITAMIN C SERUM
(15% VITAMIN C)

TIPS & TRICKS

L- Ascorbic Acid Powder is the only pure and natural form of Vitamin C that can be used safely on the skin. It absorbs easily, however, be sure to do a small test patch first as it can be irritating to those with sensitive skin. Once the skin has absorbed the powder it stimulates the creation of collagen and is a highly potent antioxidant.

You can purchase capsules and use a needle to puncture it and squeeze the liquid out.

It is best to use a dark opaque glass bottle for storage.

Do not use any kind of metal utensils during the preparation and making of the serum - only glass, wood or ceramic.

You can omit the glycerin and Vitamin E if you wish, however, the mixture will be prone to oxidation which will reduce the shelf life to 2 days.

The serum will last for up to 5 days in the fridge.

INGREDIENTS

1 teaspoon of L-Ascorbic Acid Powder
1 teaspoon of glycerin

3 teaspoons of pure distilled filtered water
¼ teaspoon of Vitamin E

DIRECTIONS

In a small nonmetal bowl add 1 teaspoon of L-Ascorbic acid to 3 teaspoons of filtered water and gently stir. Leave for 45 minutes, stirring occasionally until the crystals have dissolved. Be sure not to expose the mixture to heat as this will destroy the vital ingredients in the serum.

Once the L-ascorbic acid has dissolved add 1 teaspoon of glycerine and ¼ teaspoon Vitamin E to the mixture and stir gently.

Carefully transfer the mixture into an opaque glass container and store in the fridge for 3-5 days.

Give the mixture a good shake before each use.

HOW TO USE VITAMIN C SERUM

L-Ascorbic acid will stay active on your skin for up to 72 hours so you should not apply the serum every day. It is recommended you apply a small amount every 1-2 days for best results.

Apply to dry skin using a cotton pad or clean fingers after you have cleansed and removed all makeup. Leave the serum on for around 30 minutes before rinsing off. You may continue with the remainder of your skincare regime after you have rinsed the serum off.

ANTI-AGING CUCUMBER & ALOE FACE MASK

WHAT THIS MASK WILL DO FOR YOUR SKIN:

Cucumber: Reduces water retention and swelling in the skin, as well as reducing puffiness under the eyes. Nourishes and cleanses skin.

Aloe Vera: Natural moisturiser and reduces flakiness or dry patches.

Rose Water: Packed with vitamins and antioxidants which help prevent the signs of aging.

Lemon Juice: Packed with vitamin C to help brighten skin. Natural skin detoxifier and pore minimiser.

INGREDIENTS

¼ cup whole organic cucumber, peeled

1 Tbsp natural aloe vera gel

1 tbsp whole organic lemon, juiced

½ tsp pure rose water

DIRECTIONS

Combine all ingredients in a food processor and pulse until it becomes a smooth paste.

Wash face with warm water, ensuring all makeup is removed. Pat dry to remove excess moisture.

Apply mask to moist skin and leave for 25 minutes.

Gently remove the mask with tepid water.

Apply toner or moisturiser once skin is clean.

For best results use this mask 1-2 times per week.

BEAUTY BOOSTING BLUEBERRY & OAT EXFOLIATING MASK

WHAT THIS MASK WILL DO FOR YOUR SKIN:

Raw Almonds: High in Vitamin E and essential fatty acids

Blueberries: High in antioxidants. Rich in Vitamin C which naturally boosts collagen levels in the skin.

Oats: Anti-inflammatory properties. Acts as a gentle exfoliant and contains zinc and copper to smooth wrinkles.

Honey: Brightens skin with it's antioxidants and antibacterial properties

Milk: Cleanses skin

INGREDIENTS

¼ cup fresh organic blueberries
¼ cup whole raw almonds
1 tablespoon organic honey

2 tablespoons whole rolled oats
(do not use quick oats)
1 tablespoon whole organic milk

DIRECTIONS

Add all ingredients to a food processor and pulse until smooth. Add more milk if the mixture is too thick. The consistency should be similar to a thick cream.

Wash and cleanse skin, ensuring all makeup has been removed and gently pat skin to remove excess moisture.

Apply mask generously all over moist skin and neck and leave for 20 minutes. The mask should have dried onto your skin after 20 minutes.

In a gentle circular motion massage the mixture with clean fingers to exfoliate until it crumbles off the skin.

Remove with lukewarm water. You may follow with your skincare regime after by using a toner or a moisturiser.

For best results use once a week.

WRINKLE REDUCING BLACKBERRY & WALNUT SCRUB

WHAT THIS MASK WILL DO FOR YOUR SKIN:

Blackberries: High in antioxidants and packed full of vitamin A, C and E.

Walnuts: Good source of vitamin E. The skin of the walnut will act as an exfoliant.

INGREDIENTS

½ cup walnuts (with skin)

½ cup fresh organic blackberries (can be substituted for other dark berries)

DIRECTIONS

Add walnuts and berries to a food processor and combine until a smooth paste is formed. If the mixture is too dry or sticky add 1 tsp water at a time until desired texture is achieved.

Wash skin with tepid water and ensure all makeup has been removed. Add mask to moistened skin and exfoliate gently for a 2-3 minutes in a circular motion.

Leave mask on face and neck for an additional 3 minutes then rinse off with lukewarm water. Gently pat skin dry with a clean towel and continue with skincare regime by using toner or moisturiser.

SKIN BRIGHTENING HONEY & OATMEAL FACE MASK

WHAT THIS MASK WILL DO FOR YOUR SKIN:

Honey: Brightens skin with its antioxidants and antibacterial properties.

Oats: Anti-inflammatory properties. Acts as a gentle exfoliant and contains zinc and copper to smooth wrinkles.

INGREDIENTS

2 tablespoons organic honey

2 tablespoons rolled oats (do not use quick oats)

DIRECTIONS

Add honey and oats to a nonmetallic bowl and stir till combined.

Wash face with warm water, ensuring all makeup is removed.

Apply mask to moist skin and leave for 20 minutes.

The mask should have dried after 20 minutes. Gently remove mask by gently rubbing in a circular motion to exfoliate. Rinse residue off skin with tepid water.

Apply toner or moisturiser once skin is clean.

DETOXIFYING PAPAYA & GREEK YOGURT FACE MASK

WHAT THIS MASK WILL DO FOR YOUR SKIN:

Papaya: High in 'papain' which helps skin glow by removing dead skin cells.

Greek Yogurt: Rich in protein and lactic acid which helps tighten pores.

Lemon Juice: Packed with vitamin C to help brighten skin. Natural skin detoxifier and pore minimiser.

INGREDIENTS

¼ cup raw papaya
1 tablespoon lemon juice

2 tablespoons natural Greek yoghurt

DIRECTIONS

Add papaya, lemon and yoghurt to a food processor and pulse till smooth. Alternatively you can use a spoon to mush the ingredients together in a nonmetallic bowl and stir till combined.

Wash face with warm water, ensuring all makeup is removed.

Apply mask to moist skin and leave for 20 minutes.

Gently remove the mask with tepid water.

Apply toner or moisturiser once skin is clean.

SKIN FIRMING COCONUT OIL, EGG WHITE & STRAWBERRY FACE MASK

WHAT THIS MASK WILL DO FOR YOUR SKIN:

Egg Whites: Tightens and firms skin

Coconut Oil: Antibacterial, antifungal and antimicrobial properties to nourish skin.

Strawberries: Reduce the appearance of fine lines. High in Antibacterial properties that will clean pores and help reduce acne.

INGREDIENTS

¼ cup raw strawberries
1 egg white

1 tablespoon organic coconut oil

DIRECTIONS

Use a spoon to mash the strawberries into a puree in a nonmetallic bowl. Add egg white and coconut oil and stir till combined.

Wash face with warm water, ensuring all makeup is removed.

Apply mask to moist skin and leave for 10 minutes.

Gently remove mask with tepid water.

Apply toner or moisturiser once skin is clean.

HOMEMADE 'MIRACLE' NIGHT CREAM

WHAT THIS CREAM WILL DO FOR YOUR SKIN:

Beeswax: Forms a film to protect your skin from environmental damage. Locks in moisture and is high in Vitamin A.

Raw Shea Butter: Nourishes and moisturises skin. Protects from free radicals.

Coconut Oil: Antibacterial, antifungal and antimicrobial properties will nourish skin.

Almond Oil: Potent anti-aging properties. Removes water retention reducing puffiness under the eyes.

Lemon Oil: Packed with vitamin C to help brighten skin. Natural skin detoxifier and pore minimiser.

Vitamin E: Slows down natural aging process and helps heal scars or skin issues.

INGREDIENTS

½ tsp beeswax
1 tablespoon organic coconut oil
2 tablespoons almond oil
½ tsp of shea butter (can be substitute for coconut oil)
¼ cup aloe vera gel

1 tsp vitamin E oil (you can purchase capsules and use a needle to puncture it and squeeze the liquid out)
1 tsp organic honey
5-10 drops lemon essential oil

DIRECTIONS

In a small saucepan add beeswax, coconut oil, almond oil and shea butter. Heat gently on a low heat until melted and set aside to completely cool.

Mix together aloe vera gel, vitamin E oil, lemon oil and honey.

Combine beeswax mixture and aloe vera mixture in a blender until fully combined and it becomes the consistency of a rich cream. Add 1 tsp more coconut oil if it is too thick.

Transfer to a nonmetallic container and seal the lid. Store in a cool dry place, out of direct sunlight and use within 10 days.

Be sure not to use metallic utensils or saucepans when preparing the cream.

Use once a day in the evening after washing and cleansing your face with warm water.

ANTI-AGING MOISTURIZING DAY CREAM

WHAT THIS MASK WILL DO FOR YOUR SKIN:

Lanolin: Provides a surge of moisture, forms a protective layer over skin and has a cushioning and plumping effect.

Avocado Oil: Smoothes wrinkles, packed with vitamins A, B, D, E, K, high in antioxidants and penetrates the skin deeply. Great for smoothing out fine lines.

Wheat Germ Oil: Nutrient-packed, great at softening and moisturizing your skin

Rose Water: High in antioxidants, combats aging and packed full of vitamins.

Vitamin E: Slows down natural aging process and helps heal scars or skin issues.

Almond Oil: Potent anti-aging properties. Removes water retention reducing puffiness under the eyes.

INGREDIENTS

2 tablespoons rose water
¼ cup avocado oil
2 tablespoons almond oil
4 teaspoons wheat germ oil
2 tablespoons lanolin

2 teaspoons vegetable glycerin
¼ teaspoon retinol serum
1 capsule vitamin E, 400 IU
3 drops geranium essential oil

DIRECTIONS

In a non-metallic saucepan gently heat the rose water on a low temperature - ensuring it does not boil.

While the rose water is heating combine avocado oil, almond oil and wheat germ oil in a glass measuring cup. Fill a saucepan with around 2 inches of water and place glass cup in water. Heat over medium-low until the water is simmering.

Immediately reduce heat and add lanolin. Once lanolin has fully melted pour in rose water very slowly while whisking constantly.

Remove from heat and whisk the ingredients vigorously until you achieve a thick creamy texture.

Add vegetable glycerin, retinol serum, geranium oil and vitamin E to the mixture, stirring until all ingredients have combined.

Pour into a non-metallic pot or container and allow to cool to room temperature before securing the lid.

The cream will keep for around 2 weeks. Store in a cool dry place out of direct sunlight.

DAILY ANTI-AGING SKIN CARE REGIME

MORNING

Wash face with water and a gentle, water-soluble cleanser to remove dirt, oil, and makeup. Ensure the cleanser is suitable for your skin type (dry, oily or normal). If showering, try to have the water as cool as possible as hot showers are not good for your skin.

Apply toner using a cotton wool pad for softer and smoother skin. Toners will help reduce redness and eliminate any dry patches.

Exfoliate skin with facial scrub (preferably homemade). Do not exfoliate more than once a week and be sure to be very gentle on the skin. It is best to exfoliate with clean damp skin and apply the scrub using a gentle circular motion. Rinse off with warm water and pat dry with a clean towel.

After cleaning skin either with daily cleanser or weekly exfoliating scrub, apply day face cream. It is recommended to apply vitamin C serum once a week - for best results do this after exfoliating.

Allow face cream to absorb into skin then apply SPF 30. Even if it is over-cast or cloudy the UV rays can still penetrate the skin causing damage.

Apply moisturizing lip treatment.

EVENING

Remove all makeup using a cleanser, then wash face with lukewarm water and face soap.

Apply night cream to damp clean skin in a gentle circular motion.

Once a week apply retinol serum (not on the same day you apply Vitamin C serum).

If you spot any visible flakiness, apply Vaseline directly onto the dry patches.

Apply vaseline or moisturiser on lips.

AFTERTHOUGHT

When it comes to skincare and beauty practices, there is definitely no 'one size fits all' approach, but good and healthy practices will ensure you enjoy the fountain of youth for years to come!